MORE THAN WHAT YOU SEE

STRENGTH & DIGNITY

Alzheimer's and Me

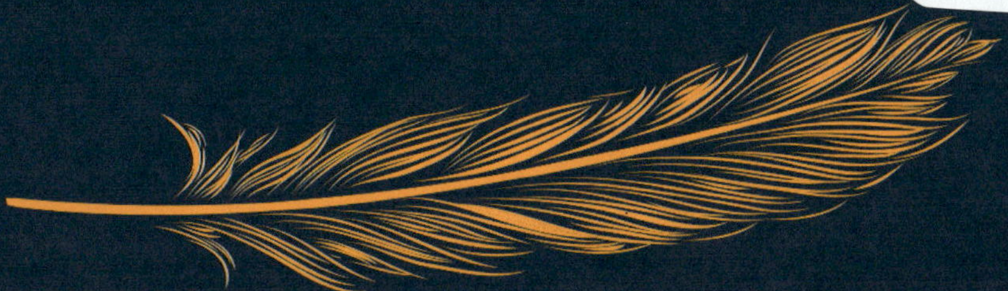

Memory Changes, but Never the Heart

Honoring the Strength that Still Shines Within

A.T. YOUNG

Copyright

Title book: STRENGTH & DIGNITY
Subtitle: Alzheimer's and Me
Author: A.T. Young
Illustrations: A.T. Young
Published by Thinking Spirit Press

www.thinkingspirit.com
First edition 2025

For more information, please contact:

author@thinkingspirit.com

Thank you for your support

Dedicated to my son, Jake.

STILL ME

You may see moments when I pause,
and lose my place without a cause.

But look again, I'm still right here,
with love to give and heart sincere.

I walk through days both calm and strange,
my world may shift, my thoughts may change.

Yet still I shine in what I do,
a life of meaning, strong and true.

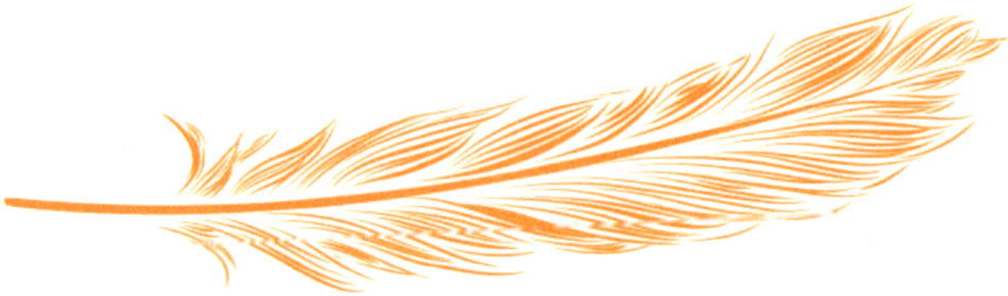

I am still me.
My worth
never fades.

FINDING CALM

My thoughts may wander, drift away,
then circle back another day.

But in the quiet, I still know,
familiar comforts help me grow.

I may forget the words to speak,
but feelings last, both strong and deep.

For though the mind may lose its track,
the heart remembers, looking back.

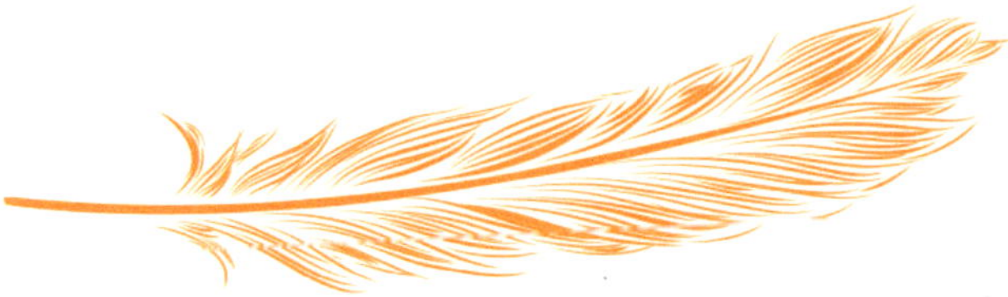

I am understood
beyond the
words I say.

THINGS CHANGE

I’m thinking life has slowed its pace,
but left behind a deeper grace.

I'm thinking some things work anew,
and I adapt the way I do.

I'm thinking change need not define
the thoughts and feelings that are mine.

I'm thinking though some things depart,
what matters most stays in my heart.

I remain
myself, even
as life changes.

WHAT REMAINS

Some think I've faded, lost my place,
a shadow with a different face.

But I'm still here, please see me clear,
I'm still myself, with much held dear.

They may not know the depth I feel,
or how familiar voices heal.

For I am more than what they see,
there's still a shining part of me.

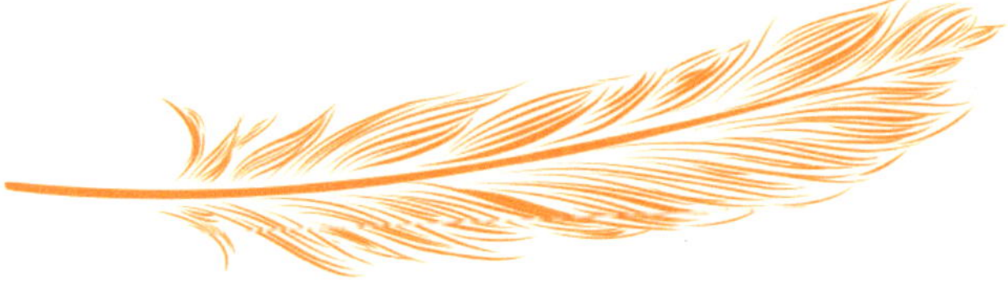

I am more than
my memory.
I am whole.

WHAT HELPS

I deal with issues day by day,
with gentle help along the way.

I lean on love, I take my rest,
and give each moment all my best.

When tasks are hard, I don't despair,
I take it slow, with steady care.

And even when my steps are small,
I still find purpose through it all.

I can accept
support and still
be myself.

MORE THAN SEEN

I should not fear the times I stray,
but find new paths along the way.

I should accept the help I need,
and trust myself with every deed.

I should remember I'm not less,
though moments bring me weariness.

I should look past what others see,
and hold on to the whole of me.

Others may
see my challenges.
I know there is more to me.

MY VOICE

A gentle hand, a smiling face,
the comfort of a warm embrace.

The songs I love, the scents I know,
the memories that still can glow.

To share a laugh, to spend some time,
and know these moments still are mine.

These simple gifts can help me stay,
connected to each passing day.

The things
I enjoy are part
of who I am.

STEP BY STEP

I carry on by walking slow,
accepting all the love I know.

I carry on by holding near,
the ones whose presence brings me cheer.

I carry on with patience true,
with all the things I still can do.

For every step, though small it be,
still leads me where I need to be.

I move
forward in my
own way.

SMALL JOYS

I've learned that slowing down is kind,
and brings more comfort to my mind.

I've learned a smile can warm the day,
in simple, unexpected ways.

I've learned that joy can still be found,
in gentle moments all around.

I've learned that though some memories fade,
my worth and value never trade.

Joy can

still be found in

everyday moments.

KEEP GOING

I'll take my rest, I'll take my time,
I'll hold to moments that are mine.

I'll treasure kindness, soft and true,
the gentle things that see me through.

I'll let the sunshine warm my face,
I'll find my comfort, find my place.

I'll meet each morning as it comes,
and value all that day becomes.

Each new
day brings something
worthwhile.

STILL GROWING

I'll share my smile, my hand, my care,
to show that warmth is always there.

I'll teach through patience, calm and grace,
the lessons time cannot erase.

I'll help remind both friends and kin,
that growth can still be found within.

For in the love I give and show,
I help another's spirit grow.

I still
have something
valuable to share.

I BELONG

You stand beside me, day by day,
guiding me along the way.

Your care is steady, calm and true,
and means far more than words can do.

But don't forget, you matter too,
this journey also touches you.

Take time to breathe, to laugh, to live,
for you deserve the love you give.

We stay
connected through
care and understanding.

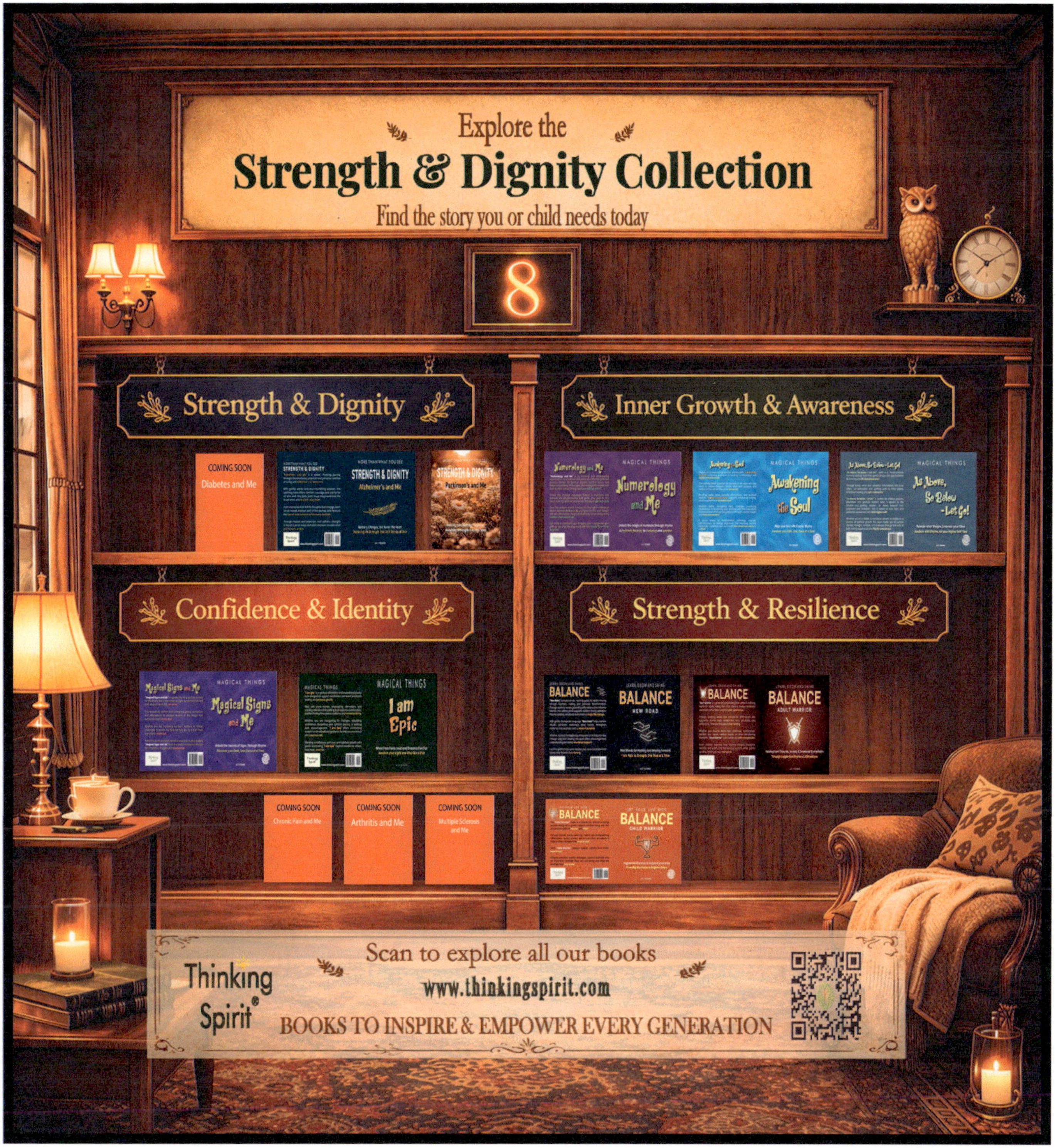
Explore the
Strength & Dignity Collection
Find the story you or child needs today
8
Strength & Dignity
COMING SOON
Diabetes and Me
STRENGTH & DIGNITY
Alzheimer's and Me
STRENGTH & DIGNITY
Parkinson's and Me
Inner Growth & Awareness
MAGICAL THINGS
Numerology and Me
MAGICAL THINGS
Awakening the Soul
MAGICAL THINGS
As Above, So Below - Let Go!
Confidence & Identity
MAGICAL THINGS
Magical Signs and Me
MAGICAL THINGS
I am Epic
Strength & Resilience
BALANCE
NEW ROAD
BALANCE
ADULT WARRIOR
COMING SOON
Chronic Pain and Me
COMING SOON
Arthritis and Me
COMING SOON
Multiple Sclerosis and Me
BALANCE
CHILD WARRIOR
Scan to explore all our books
Thinking Spirit®
www.thinkingspirit.com
BOOKS TO INSPIRE & EMPOWER EVERY GENERATION

Please use the blank pages in this book for your own thoughts, memories, reflections, or messages to those you love.

Thank you for reading and sharing this journey.

If you found this book meaningful, please consider leaving an Amazon review. Your review helps others find this book and the message it shares.

Made in the USA
Monee, IL
05 November 2026

67382334R00019